MW01300027

Anti-Inflammatory Eating Plan (AIEP)

A Four-Week Journey

Sharon Graham, R.N.

www.TheCoachingPair.com

JIREH Marketing, Inc.

Copyright Notice

Copyright © 2012 by JIREH Marketing, Inc. All Rights Reserved.

Reproduction or translation of any part of this work beyond that permitted by section 107 or 108 of the 1976 United States Copyright Act without permission of the copyright owner is unlawful. Requests for permission or further information should be addressed to the author.

Sharon Graham, R.N., JIREH Marketing, Inc.
421 Currituck Drive, Chesapeake, VA, 23322, USA
www.TheCoachingPair.com

Any and all information contained herein is not intended to take the place of medical advice from a healthcare professional. This information is for educational and informational purposes only. Readers should always consult with a physician before taking any actions of any kind relating to their health. The author nor publisher will in no way be held responsible for any reader who fails to do so. Any action taken based on these contents is at the sole discretion and liability of the reader.

First Printing, 2012

ISBN-13: 978-1475059144

ISBN-10: 1475059140

Printed in the United States of America

Table of Contents

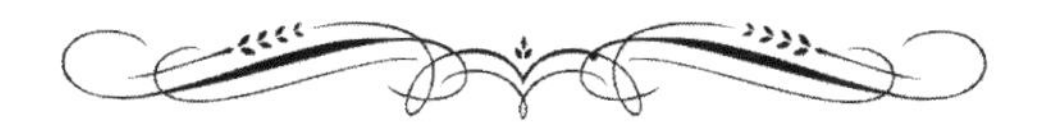

Preface

The contents of this book were originally presented as a series of daily blog posts on our blog, www.TheCoachingPair.com/blog.

The Coaching Pair Blog

As such it is essentially a daily diary or journal covering our experiences over a period of four weeks during which we "walked our talk" and ate according to a plan I created from reading a multitude of sources.

Given that understanding of the genesis of this book, please excuse the rather unconventional formatting and seeming repetition. Remember, it's a day-by-day accounting of my thoughts and experiences as we walked through some unfamiliar territory. I wrestled with the notion of reformatting to a more traditional book presentation, but rejected the idea because it seemed that some of the power of the journal format would be lost.

The idea to create a book from previously published blog posts is to satisfy the demand by more recent clients who need the information, but who weren't following The Coaching Pair when it was originally written. Thank you for your understanding.

Warmly,
Coach Sharon

PS – The funny looking little black and white squares (e.g., on the previous page) that are used in selected places throughout this book are two-dimensional bar codes, called quick response codes (QR codes). Think of them as paper-based hyperlinks. You simply take a picture of a QR code with your smart phone, and you get redirected to a website using your cell phone's browser. Much, much easier and faster than trying to type a long web site url into your browser without making a mistake.

Also, all the photos in this book were taken and saved with the Internet in mind. As you probably know, photo resolution requirements for the Internet are considerably lower than for a printed book such as this. Frankly, the printed photos looked ghastly, so the QR codes will allow you to view the photos in a much more appetizing manner.

Introduction Inflammation: The Real Killer

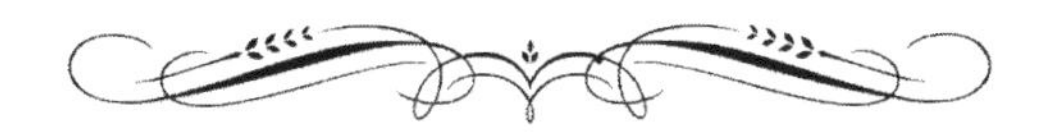

Inflammation is a HOT topic. [pun intended] Most of the nutrition newsletters, magazines, and articles I'm reading touch on the subject of inflammation. Just doing a quick Internet search on inflammation brought up 63,600,000 entries!

Disorders and diseases such as arthritis, MS, fibromyalgia, osteoporosis, diabetes, and even obesity are correlated with chronic inflammation within the body. Today's many chemical exposures along with the modern diet and lifestyle are the main contributors to this "smoldering situation."

I became more intrigued about the correlation of diet and inflammation after reading the (then newly published) life-altering book by Dr. Jordan Rubin titled *The Maker's Diet.*

The Maker's Diet
(http://jireh.us/MakersDiet)

I've since coached dozens of people using his program which is specifically designed to stabilize blood sugar levels, balance hormone levels, improve digestion, and REDUCE INFLAMMATION.

Granted there are now many anti-inflammatory "diet programs" out there. However, through reading and researching numerous respected authors, I've discovered common ground on the predominant, inflammatory causing foods.

Dr. Russell Blaylock hits hard on the excitotoxic food additives such as MSG, hydrolyzed proteins, autolyzed yeast, etc., and the "pro-inflammatory" fats such as corn, safflower, sunflower, peanut, soybean, and canola oils. Trans fats such as margarine and any and all fried foods are also extremely detrimental.

Refined carbohydrates such as white bread, rolls, pastries, crackers, etc. all cause systemic inflammation. It should go without saying, but to set the record straight, all fast-food and/or drive-through food will contribute to inflammation in a major way. White refined sugar along with all artificial sweeteners is also pro-inflammatory.

Dr. Joseph Mercola began talking about the inflammatory effects of grains many years ago. It's not a popular subject as people love their breads, cereals, and pasta. On Dr. Rubin's program, there are no grains in the first few weeks.

Jerry and I personally have done The Maker's Diet program several times before. And even though we both eat a healthy, clean diet, we're feeling the need/desire to embrace a more specific anti-inflammatory eating plan for a few weeks. Therefore,

I'm taking pieces of a few programs and designing our own anti-inflammatory program.

I'd like to invite you to join us. If you're plagued with aches and pains, or with excess pounds that you don't want, or just want to feel better and accelerate your health journey, embark on this with us. I've decided to post blogs on what we're eating each day and what we're noticing with regard to our energy and overall health.

For further info on the effects of inflammation, see the following great article:

Inflammation Illnesses
(http://jireh.us/illnesslist)

Anti-Inflammatory Eating Plan (AIEP)

As promised, we're starting a multi-week eating plan (instead of a DIE-t) which I'm choosing to call AIEP or Anti-Inflammatory Eating Plan. Every day, we will post a short update of what we ate the day before.

The AIEP is not designed for weight loss. However, if your body needs to shed some fat, it is highly probable that that will happen. If you are already thin and don't want or need to lose weight, then have frequent snacks of almonds and walnuts and make smoothies with coconut milk and berries.

Here is what we'll be eating for the first two weeks:

Meats

I have some of the first three in the freezer:

--Grass-fed beef

--Buffalo

--Venison

You could also eat lamb or veal but Jerry doesn't really care for either.

Poultry

Free range, no hormones or antibiotics

--Chicken

--Turkey

--Nitrate free turkey bacon (Applegate Farms is the brand I have)

--Free range, organic eggs (I get ours from a local farmer)

Fish

--Salmon, wild-caught salmon that I have in the freezer. I also bought some wild-caught canned salmon for use in salads.

--Roughy, Halibut, and Cod, all wild-caught

Dairy

--Organic, unsalted butter (Trader Joe's is a fair price.)

--Plain goat milk yogurt

--Soft goat cheese

No other dairy for the first two weeks

Fats

--Organic, extra virgin olive oil for salads

--Organic coconut oil for cooking

--Avocadoes

--Organic unsalted butter as mentioned above

--Coconut milk (in a can; no sulfites)

Nuts

--Raw almonds, soaked and dried as in the following article:

Easy to digest nuts
(http://jireh.us/nuts)

--Raw walnuts, soaked and dried as above
--Raw sunflower seeds (I soak these as well but not totally necessary, they taste better though.)
--Raw pumpkin seeds, soaked in salt water with cayenne pepper, dried as above
--Flax seeds (ground); I prefer golden flax seeds
--Hemp seeds
--Chia seeds
--Raw almond butter
--Tahini (sesame butter)

Fruits

--Blueberries
--Blackberries
--Raspberries
--Strawberries
--Lemons
--Limes

Vegetables

--Broccoli
--Brussels sprouts
--Cabbage
--Cauliflower
--Carrots
--Green beans
--Onions
--Romaine lettuce
--Spring mix and all lettuces except iceberg
--Spinach
--Summer squash
--Zucchini
--Beets
--Celery

--Cucumbers
--Mushrooms
--Peppers
--Tomatoes
--Leafy greens such as kale and collards
--Peas
--Asparagus
--Eggplant
--Garlic

Beans

--Lentils
--Miso (fermented soybean paste)

Condiments

Mine are all organic without preservatives, MSG, sugar or high fructose corn syrup

--Salsa
--Tomato sauce
--Ketchup
--Mustard
--Vegenaise (Purple lid; made with grapeseed oil). No mayonnaise is perfect but I prefer this over one made from soybean oil)
--Tamari (wheat free soy sauce)
--Herbamare (sea salt with herbs)
--Apple cider vinegar
--Sea salt
--Balsamic vinegar
--Brown rice vinegar
--Umeboshi vinegar
--Vanilla extract

Sweeteners

--2 tablespoons of raw honey per day

I may use small amounts of stevia if needed to make a dressing palatable

Beverages

--Purified, filtered water (half of your body weight in ounces per day)

--Organic herbal teas

--Raw green juices with 1 or 2 carrots added for flavor (made fresh with juicer)

--Kombucha, plain.

Week 1 – Day 1 Results

Yesterday we began our AIEP (Anti-Inflammatory Eating Plan). I've read and studied various books and articles on inflammation by several different authors. I've taken what I believe to be the best information from several sources and devised a plan that I think is quite doable for anyone who is ready to take their health to the next level.

Instead of looking at the foods that aren't on the AIEP list, look and embrace ALL of the wonderful God-given foods that you ***can*** eat and enjoy! I should reiterate that this is what Jerry and I are choosing to do. And even though I believe this to be a very healthful and sound eating plan, please understand that I can take no responsibility for anyone else.

Again, this eating plan is designed to stabilize blood sugar levels, balance hormone levels, improve digestion, and REDUCE INFLAMMATION. Here is what we ate on Day 1.

Breakfast

--Sautéed onion, orange pepper, and mushrooms in coconut oil until soft. Added fresh spinach and sautéed until wilted. Added eggs, cayenne and Herbamare and cooked lightly.

--Fresh strawberries

Snack

--Almonds

Lunch

--Large salad with fresh lettuce from a friend's garden topped with cucumbers, radishes, grape tomatoes, orange pepper, avocado, goat cheese, and sunflower seeds.

--Dressing of olive oil, balsamic vinegar and herbs

--Blackberries

Snack

--Almonds

Dinner

--Ground beef meatloaf made with lots of vegetables such as onion, garlic, red pepper, carrot, zucchini and herbs.

--Steamed broccoli w/butter

--Raw salad of red pepper, avocado, cucumber, onion, tomato, walnuts w/oil and vinegar dressing and herbs.

Meatloaf Dinner Photo
(http://jireh.us/1-1)

Snack

--Coconut milk w/frozen mixed berries (blended in the Magic Bullet)

Week 1 – Day 2 Results

Here is what we ate on Day 2.
(Yesterday was church day so breakfast had to be less time consuming. Saturday's breakfast was simple but it did take a little more time with the cutting up of the vegetables.)

Breakfast

--I placed frozen mixed berries in a large bowl when I got up so they could partially thaw. When ready to eat, I added ground flax seeds, hemp seeds, sunflower seeds and goat yogurt with a tiny drizzle of raw honey. Stirred that together and it was very yummy. Filling too. No snack since we were in church.

Lunch

--We ate more of a dinner menu having leftover meatloaf and steamed broccoli. Green salad with spring mix and leftover vegetable salad from Saturday evening spooned on top.

--Fresh strawberries

Snack

--Pumpkin seeds and almonds

Supper

--We usually just snack on Sunday evenings. We ate raw carrots and celery with almond butter and some soft herbed goat cheese.

--Walnuts and blackberries

--Later on I mixed coconut milk, frozen blueberries and a tiny drizzle (1/2 teaspoon) of honey in Magic Bullet.

Week 1 – Day 3 Results

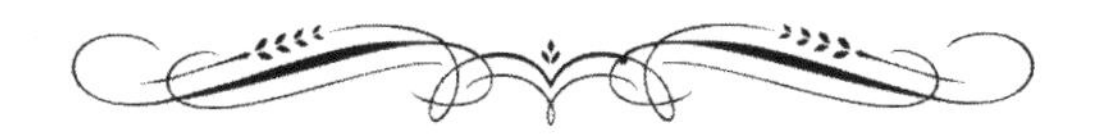

Here is what we ate on Day 3.

Breakfast

(We went to the gym and hurried home as I had a Skype call scheduled for first thing. However, I was surprised at how little time it took to make this wonderfully healthy meal.)

--I sautéed onions, mushrooms, and peppers in coconut oil. (It really only took minutes to cut up the mushrooms, onion and pepper.) Then I added a handful of fresh spinach and let it wilt. Next I added 6 eggs and some soft goat cheese. I cooked the eggs very gently and very little. Yummo!

--Ate some fresh blackberries afterward.

Snack

Blackberries

Lunch

--Large salad with spring mix, peppers, avocado, cucumber, tomatoes, goat cheese, and sunflower seeds. Olive oil, balsamic vinegar and herb dressing.

Snack

--Almonds

--Pumpkin seeds

Dinner

--I thawed frozen chicken breasts (with bone). Put almond meal (ground almonds) in a baggie. Added paprika, garlic powder, Herbamare, parsley and lemon thyme. Melted butter in glass 13 x 9 inch baking dish. Placed each breast in bag and coated with mixture. Placed in baking dish. Baked at 350 degrees.

--Marinated cut up zucchini and yellow summer squash in olive oil, balsamic vinegar, garlic and fresh rosemary. Roasted in 350 degree oven. (Jerry was on a coaching call and we mis-communicated with one another so the vegetables got a little overdone.)

--Coleslaw (Grated cabbage, broccoli, and carrots; dressing of Vegenaise, apple cider vinegar, and Herbamare). I thought the slaw might need a bit of stevia, however it was fine with the Vegenaise and vinegar.

Almond-Baked Chicken Dinner Photo
(http://jireh.us/1-3a)

Our taste buds are losing their desire for sweetness. Fresh, raw strawberries, blueberries, and blackberries are actually tasting quite sweet.

Since Jerry and I live a relatively healthy lifestyle and eat a diet of mostly organic and whole foods, I didn't know what we might experience when beginning this program. We've done something similar several times before and usually have signs of detoxification in the beginning.

I haven't necessarily noticed anything negative this time. I have noticed that I'm sleeping more soundly. I fall asleep quickly and stay asleep. I do have to go to the bathroom during the night but I fall immediately back to sleep. I had no less energy at the gym and was a bit surprised by that.

Week 1 – Day 4 Results

Here is what we ate on Day 4.

Breakfast

--I partially thawed frozen blueberries. Then added ground flax seeds, hemp seeds, almond butter, cinnamon and goat yogurt. Gently mixed it together. Although it wasn't really pretty enough for a picture, it was delicious and filling.

Snack

--Almonds

Lunch

--Leftover vegetables from last night's dinner (zucchini and summer squash) and leftover vegetable salad (avocado, cucumber, peppers, onions, and tomatoes) plus some grape tomatoes. We both had phone call appointments so the leftovers were very convenient.

Snack

--Goat cheese--this was a little more filling for a snack than just berries since our lunch was rather light.

Dinner

--I took the leftover chicken from last night and removed it from the bone. Chopped it into pieces and added chopped celery, onion, walnuts, cucumber, and red pepper. I made a dressing of Vegenaise, Dijon mustard, apple cider vinegar, Herbamare, cayenne pepper, and curry powder. Stirred it all together and served on mixed spring greens with fresh tomatoes. It was quite satisfying for both of us.

Chicken Salad Photo
(http://jireh.us/1-4)

This is a variation from how I normally make chicken salad but it was still quite good. Usually I use pecans, apples, and dried cranberries and make a little sweeter dressing. That can be eaten in a later phase of the AIEP.

We were on a training call in the evening so neither of us had a desire for a snack.

Week 1 – Day 5 Results

Here is what we ate on Day 5.

Breakfast

--Yesterday, I made us smoothies for breakfast. I used a can of coconut milk, frozen raspberries (yes, they were organic), fresh spinach (you can't taste it), eggs (yes we eat raw eggs), walnuts, Super Seed from Garden of Life, a small scoop of a green powder, and a specialty whey protein powder called OsoLean. Blended all in the blender. Thick and delicious and quite filling.

Snack

--Didn't have a desire for anything.

Lunch

--We ate leftover vegetable slaw from the other evening, leftover chicken salad, and fresh tomatoes.

--Had some fresh organic strawberries as well.

Snack

--Almonds

Dinner

--I made lentil soup with lentils (I soaked them for several hours), onion, celery, garlic, carrot, summer squash, cabbage, tomatoes, chicken broth (that I had frozen from roasting a chicken), herbs, and spices. --Had a fresh green salad as well.

Lentil Soup w/Salad Photo
(http://jireh.us/1-5)

Even though we eat a clean, healthy diet, there were still times when I wanted something sweet after a meal or between meals. I might eat a couple of dates or figs or other fruit to satisfy that desire. Some evenings I would make us a “treat” with almond butter, carob or cocoa powder, coconut, various other seeds and nuts, and either honey, agave nectar, or stevia.

I’ve realized that the desire for something sweet has not only diminished, it’s gone! I’m so satisfied with the food we’re eating that I’ve not even thought of having anything sweet.

Week 1 – Day 6 Results

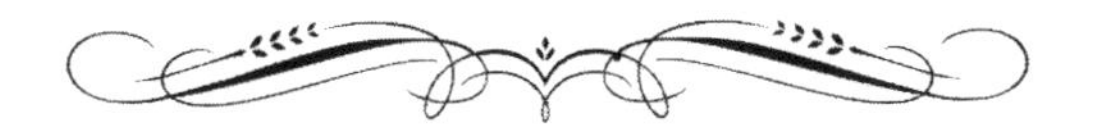

Here is what we ate on Day 6.

Breakfast & Lunch

--We fasted for breakfast and lunch yesterday with the exception of a green juice for lunch. The green juice was made with spinach, spring greens, cucumber, celery, and a couple of small carrots.

Green Juice Photo
(http://jireh.us/1-6)

Fasting used to be a regular discipline for Jerry for many years. There were a number of years that I was too ill to fast. And we've continued to do occasional fasting but not on a regular basis.

Fasting for spiritual reasons is quite common. However, there is a number of health benefits received through regular fasting. Jordan Rubin writes, "This partial-fast day allows the body to cleanse and rebuild." For another, more technical view of a partial fast, check this article by Dr. Ben Kim discussing the benefits of weekly fasting:

Fasting Benefits
(http://jireh.us/fasting)

Dinner
--For dinner we had leftover lentil soup with a green salad similar to Day 5.
Snack
--Handful of almonds

Week 1 – Day 7 Results

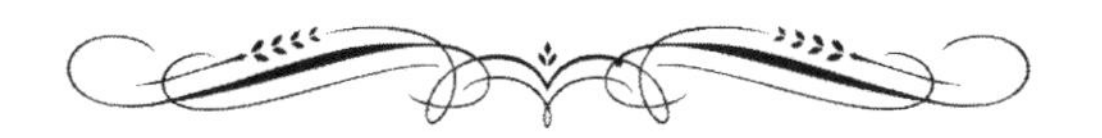

Here is what we ate on Day 7.

Breakfast

--Yesterday we had blueberries topped with ground flax seeds, hemp seeds, sunflower seeds, coconut (organic, unsweetened), almond butter, cinnamon, goat yogurt, and a tiny drizzle of raw honey.

Snack

--Almonds

Lunch

--The vegetable bin is getting low. I did have a head of cauliflower that I wanted to use. So, I cut up half of the head and added diced avocado, cucumber, red pepper, and celery. I made a dressing of Vegenaise, Dijon mustard, fresh lemon juice, celery seeds, cayenne pepper, and Herbamare. Mixed all together and served on a bed of spring mixed greens. Sprinkled with paprika.

Cauliflower-Avocado Salad Photo
(http://jireh.us/1-7)

Snack
--Freshly picked strawberries and goat cheese
Dinner
--I am blessed to be married to a man who likes leftovers. If something tastes good, I could serve it for several days in a row and Jerry would never complain. The lentil soup from a couple of days ago made a large quantity. We had it again for supper last evening.
--Spinach salad with other fresh vegetables accompanied the soup.

Week 2 – Day 8 Results

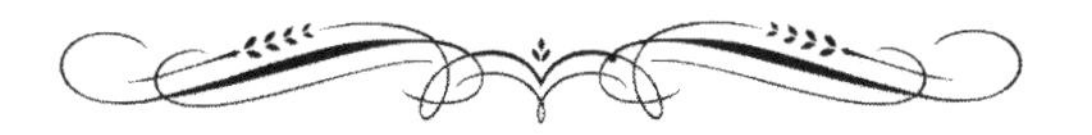

Here is what we ate on Day 8.

Breakfast

--We had a luscious smoothie using coconut milk, eggs, and fresh strawberries. Yummo and it didn't even need any sweetener.

Snack

--Almonds

Lunch

--I had lentils cooked from earlier this week when I made lentil soup. So, I made lentil burgers with the lentils, chopped onion, celery, carrot, parsley, and walnuts.

Lentil Burgers Photo
(http://jireh.us/2-8)

I added eggs, tomato paste, almond meal, and herbs such as cayenne, dry mustard, and Herbamare. I pan sautéed them in coconut oil. They didn't stick together like a meat burger, but I was able to turn them and each side browned nicely. Served on a bed of lettuce with fresh tomato and Vegenaise.

Snack

--Strawberries and goat cheese

Dinner

--Sautéed onion and garlic in coconut oil; added fresh kale, chicken broth, and crushed red pepper flakes. Cooked briefly until kale was wilted. Stirred in miso.

--Pan sautéed yellow summer squash in coconut oil and butter. Added seasonings.

--Fresh green salad

--Fresh strawberries for dessert

Yesterday made one week of our anti-inflammatory eating plan. We've had ample energy. We worked outside yesterday and felt a "good tired" when we went to bed.

We'll continue with this plan for another week, and then next weekend we'll add some other foods to the list.

Week 2 – Day 9 Results

Here is what we ate on Day 9.

Breakfast

--Church day, so we had fresh strawberries, ground flax seeds, hemp seeds, coconut, goat yogurt, and a drizzle of raw honey.

By the way, for those who think they could never acquire a taste for goat yogurt, I would offer a challenge to you. When mixed with ingredients such as those listed above, and if the yogurt is fresh, I believe it's possible that you wouldn't even recognize the goat yogurt. Just a thought.

Snack

--While preparing lunch we snacked on almonds.

Lunch

--We each had a lentil burger left over from Saturday.

--We had a spinach salad.

--We also had fresh, green beans, lightly steamed. I added olive oil, garlic, Ume Plum vinegar, a pinch of cayenne pepper, and freshly diced tomatoes to the beans. Gently stirred them together and garnished with walnuts (that had been soaked and dried).

Green Beans Photo
(http://jireh.us/2-9)

Dinner

--I bought an eggplant last week in hopes of making something special with it. I realized I needed to use it and really didn't want to spend hours fixing a dish. So, I made baba ghanoush. I roasted the eggplant in the oven, allowed it to cool and then peeled it and mashed the flesh. I then added tahini (sesame butter), garlic, lemon juice, cumin, cayenne, parsley, salt, and olive oil. We dipped fresh vegetables with it.

Snack

--Fresh blackberries

I realize we've had some meatless meals here lately. I didn't purposely plan on eating as a "vegetabletarian," as Jerry says. I guess I cooked so many lentils and made so much lentil soup that we had leftovers a number of days. I'm also the daughter of two parents who lived through the depression, so I have a challenge with letting food go to waste. I'll plan on chicken and salmon this week.

We'll remain with this eating plan until the weekend and then I'll add some new fruits, vegetables, nuts, and beans for the next two weeks.

Week 2 – Day 10 Results

Here is what we ate on Day 10.

Breakfast

--Busy morning; blueberries, ground flax seeds, hemp seeds, almond butter, goat yogurt, dash of cinnamon, vanilla extract, and a drizzle of raw honey.

Snack

--Almonds

Lunch

--Large green salad with fresh lettuce from a friend's garden, cucumbers, tomatoes, goat cheese, and sunflower seeds.

Snack

--Pumpkin seeds

Dinner

--Pan-seared salmon with a sauce of garlic, ginger, tamari, brown rice vinegar, and sesame seeds.

--Pea salad with peas, celery, cucumber, onion, goat cheese, olive oil, and brown rice vinegar dressing with herbs and spices.

--Slaw with carrots and cabbage. Dressing was olive oil, apple cider vinegar, honey, spices, and herbs.

Pan-Seared Salmon Dinner Photo
(http://jireh.us/2-10)

Even though I wouldn't say I had sleep challenges, there were times when I was restless, or would have a little difficulty falling back to sleep after getting up to go to the bathroom during the night. Since eating the AIEP, I have noticed that I sleep more soundly and deeper. Even though I do go to the bathroom during the night, the frequency has decreased and I very easily fall right back to sleep.

And again, my level of health going into this eating plan was high, but I seemed to frequently reach for a tissue to wipe or blow my nose. I realized yesterday that I'm rarely doing that. Now, I'm not saying that this AIEP has cured all ills. I'm merely sharing what I've noticed in my own person as we walk through this.

If you're walking this journey with us, please share with us what you're noticing. We can all learn from one another.

Week 2 – Day 11 Results

Here is what we ate on Day 11.

Breakfast

--Turkey bacon without nitrates from Applegate Farms.

--Eggs

--Raspberries

Lunch

--Leftover slaw

--Leftover pea salad

--Cut up avocado with garlic, lemon juice, hot pepper sauce, and soft goat cheese

Snack

--Strawberries

Dinner

--Lightly steamed kale dressed with garlic, salt, brown rice vinegar, and olive oil and tossed with fresh leaf lettuce; I topped this with a salad mixture of cauliflower, shredded carrots, sliced peppers and cucumbers mixed with olive oil and brown rice vinegar. Placed leftover cold salmon on top of that. Yummy! (This wasn't necessarily a recipe but as some of you

have probably noticed, I make up recipes with the ingredients I have on hand. I may never make this again. Or at least not the same way.)
--Blackberries

Kale Salad Topped w/Salmon Photo
(http://jireh.us/2-11)

Week 2 – Day 12 Results

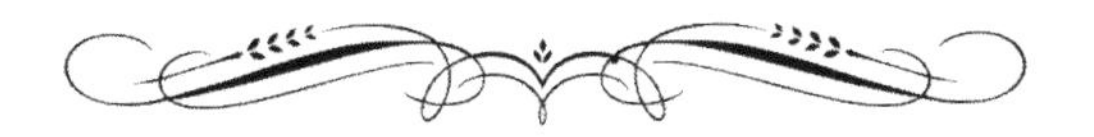

Here is what we ate on Day 12.

Breakfast

--We did our partial fasting day yesterday. I did make vegetable juice for us using greens, cucumber, parsley, celery, spinach, carrots, and an organic lemon.

Lunch

Fasting for Jerry is easy. He could go for days, without difficulty, just drinking water. Although he would say he wants something to exercise his teeth. I, on the other hand experience hunger and don't feel all that great when I go a day without some type of food.

--So for lunch, I made a green smoothie in the blender using spinach, water, ice, and various powders such as vitamin C powder, Super Seed, OsoLean powder (whey protein), and a green powder called Nitro-Greens. It wasn't sweet, thick, or necessarily smooth but it was filling and was certainly easier on the digestive system than eating a meal. Many people fast by drinking green smoothies. Even if not fasting, green smoothies are still a great way to get extra greens in our diets.

Perhaps you're wondering what the difference is between freshly made juice and smoothies. Juice is made using a juice extractor. Juices provide your body with nutrients quickly without the body having to break down and digest the whole foods. When juicing, the liquid from the fruits and vegetables is being squeezed out (extracted) and separated from the pulp or the fiber, leaving only the liquid to drink. By separating the juice from the fiber, the body is able to assimilate the nutrients quicker, allowing the digestive systems to have a rest. When we juice, we're allowing our bodies to work less and use that reserved energy to detoxify, heal and maintain our body's health.

Green smoothies, as I mentioned above, usually contain some type of greens such as spinach, kale, or romaine lettuce along with other vegetables such as celery or parsley and water and ice. They're made in a blender using the entire vegetable so they do contain fiber and pulp. Since they're blended until smooth, they too offer a rest for the digestive system; however they're not as quickly assimilated as vegetable juice. Some people put fruit in their green smoothies such as pineapple, apples, and berries.

Most people are familiar with regular smoothies that contain some type of milk or yogurt and fruit. Using frozen fruit makes them thick and well...smooth. Even though I do make smoothies with fruit, I usually always add some type of greens to add further nourishment.

Dinner

--Rather than eat a meal, we decided to just have a smoothie. This one was different than the green smoothie we had for lunch. I made this one with coconut milk, fresh strawberries, hemp seeds, and eggs. It was tasty and filling.

--We also munched on leftover vegetable salad.

We both continue to have ample and sustained energy.

Week 2 – Day 13 Results

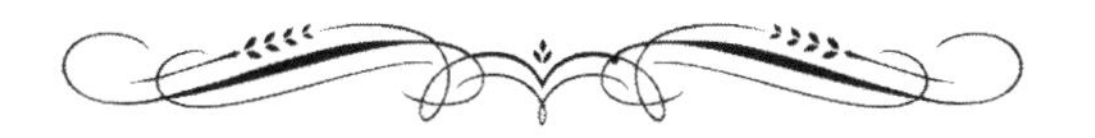

Here is what we ate on Day 13.

Breakfast

--We only had two eggs left so I made us smoothies instead of eggs. I used coconut milk, hemp seeds, blackberries, blueberries, the two eggs, spinach, mixed ascorbate powder (vitamin C powder), OsoLean powder, and Super Seed.

(By the way, if anyone is interested in having any of the Biotics products, I can offer you a referral as they only market their products through health care professionals. I had to send them my nurse's license so they would know I'm legit.)

Snack

--Almonds

Lunch

--Zucchini spaghetti

--Small green salad

Oh, this was fun! I can't take credit for the idea though. In one of my raw food cookbooks (is that an oxymoron?), I saw that they used zucchini squash as spaghetti. I know it sounds weird, but hold on. The cookbook said to use a vegetable spiral slicer. I do have one of those tools, but knew that would take longer than the time I had available.

I remembered that I have a julienne blade for my Cuisinart food processor. I first experimented with a cucumber (since I had more cucumbers than squash). After seeing how it worked with the cucumber, I was encouraged. I cut the zucchini to fit the large feeding tube of the food processor, put it in there lengthwise and pushed the button. Voila! It worked! Out came pretty, white shreds with pale green edges, very much resembling spaghetti (with green edges).

Raw Zucchini-Spaghetti Photo
(http://jireh.us/2-13)

Ideally, I would have made a raw pasta sauce or pesto. I had time for neither. I did have a jar of organic pasta sauce (with no soybean oil) to which I added herbs and spices and gently heated on top of the stove. Folks, this was delicious. Next time I'll go all out and make meatballs and the sauce to accompany the dish. But not bad for a first try.

Snack

--Raspberries

Dinner

--Large green salad with mixed greens, cucumber, peppers, onions, carrots, goat cheese, and chicken.

--Strawberries

Thank you to those of you who answered our survey question earlier in the week. The question was simply whether or not you wanted me to continue my daily updates as we move into phase 2 of the AIEP. A clear majority (almost 2/3) of you encouraged me to continue--so I shall. Thank you for your encouragement and many kind words

Week 2 – Day 14 Results

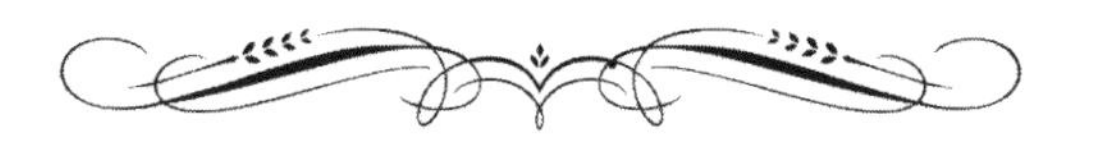

Here is what we ate on Day 14

Breakfast

--Eggs with spinach and onions

Lunch

--A large green salad topped with a fresh salad made with chopped avocado, cucumber, pepper, onion, and tomato in an olive oil and balsamic vinegar dressing. Soft goat cheese topped it off.

Green Salad w/Goat Cheese Photo
(http://jireh.us/2-14)

--Blackberries and goat yogurt. I added vanilla extract, cinnamon, and drizzle of honey to the yogurt.

Snack

--Almonds

Dinner

--Souped-up hamburgers (I added onion, parsley, Dijon mustard, tamari, garlic, almond meal, egg, and organic steak seasoning to the grass-fed beef.)

--Green beans seasoned with butter and Herbamare
--Spinach salad

Evening Snack (Date Night)

--Flax seeds, almond butter, goat yogurt, vanilla extract, and honey

Phase 2 of AIEP

We just concluded the last day of the first two weeks (Phase 1) of the AIEP. For a recap of that phase, you can go to the list of foods on page 7. We'll add some other foods for the next two weeks. Every day, and by popular demand, I will post a short update of what we ate the day before.

Remember, the AIEP is not designed for weight loss. However, if your body needs to shed some fat, it is highly probable that that will happen.

So, along with the foods listed from the first two weeks, we'll add the following:

Meats

The same meat, fish, poultry and eggs from the first two weeks.

--Sliced turkey breast (free-range, preservative free)

--Sliced roast beef (preservative free)

--Chicken or turkey sausage (nitrate free, no pork casing)

Dairy

Jerry and I are going to stay with goat milk cheese and yogurt for two more weeks. However, feel free to add:

--Organic, plain, whole milk cow's yogurt
--Organic plain kefir
--Raw cow's milk hard cheese
--Raw goat's milk
--Raw cow's milk

Fats

Same as first two weeks

Nuts

Same as first two weeks along with:
--Pecans (soaked and dried as in the following article:

Easy to digest nuts
(http://jireh.us/nuts)

Fruits

All fruits from first two weeks along with:
--Apples
--Pineapple
--Kiwi
--Pears
--Peaches
--Cantaloupe
--Plums
--Apricots
--Oranges
--Grapefruit

--Cherries

Organic is always best due to the amount of pesticides used in growing fruit. There is common agreement that the highest pesticides are found in apples, strawberries, peaches, and imported grapes.

Vegetables

Same wonderful veggies as before plus:

--Sweet Potatoes and Yams

Beans

The same as the first two weeks plus you may add:

--Pinto beans

--Black Beans

--Split Peas

--Navy Beans

Everything else is the same as the first two weeks

As I mentioned a couple of days ago, the consensus was for us to continue sharing what we eat each day.

Please know that this is not a "piece of cake" for me. I too, need to think and plan. Although we eat a relatively clean and healthy diet, this accountability has been good for me as well.

Yes, we routinely eat a fair amount of salads and vegetables; however we are eating even more of both since being on this plan. And as I've mentioned, I am sleeping deeper and sounder than I have in a long time.

I'm regularly waking up feeling refreshed and ready to go and I'm not feeling any fatigue throughout the day. Again, even though I felt well before, I believe I have an even better overall sense of well-being.

Yesterday I was able to push myself on the stair stepper at the gym unlike anything I've done before. It wasn't easy...but I did it.

Week 3 – Day 15 Results

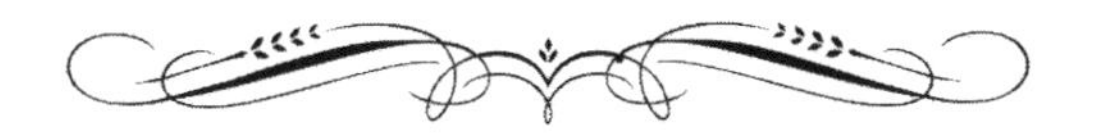

Today is the first day of the second, two weeks of the AIEP. Here is what we ate on Day 15.

Breakfast

--Green juice with greens, celery, parsley, and a couple of carrots.

--Eggs with spinach and red pepper

--Blackberries

Snack

--Almonds

Lunch

--Leftover hamburgers from the evening before.

--Small green salad

--Almost Waldorf salad; chopped apples, celery, sunflower seeds, and walnuts, but no raisins or dried cranberries. I did have fresh apricots so I cut up one of those and added it to the salad. Amazing what that little bit of sweetness did. Dressing was goat yogurt, Vegenaise, vanilla extract, cinnamon, and drizzle of honey.

Dinner

--I marinated venison pieces in tamari, olive oil, apple cider vinegar, and garlic for several hours. Removed meat from marinade and placed in the crock-pot with onions and garlic. I added tamari, cayenne pepper, and some chicken stock that I had in the refrigerator. It cooked for several hours and was fork tender when we ate it.

--Baked sweet potatoes with butter. Oh, they tasted so good!

--Small green salad

Snack

--Goat yogurt, flax seeds, blackberries, cinnamon, vanilla.

Week 3 – Day 16 Results

Instead of looking at the foods that aren't on the AIEP list, look and embrace ALL of the wonderful God-given foods that you ***can*** eat and enjoy! We are now into phase 2 of the eating plan and several foods have been added. For the list of additions, see AIEP Phase 2 on page 51.

I should reiterate that this is what Jerry and I are choosing to do. And even though I believe this to be a very healthful and sound eating plan, please understand that I can take no responsibility for anyone else.

Again, this eating plan is designed to stabilize blood sugar levels, balance hormone levels, improve digestion, and REDUCE INFLAMMATION. Here is what we ate on Day 16.

Breakfast

--Church day so we ate fresh fruit: pineapple, apricots, and blackberries, and goat yogurt.

Snack

--Snacked on almonds while preparing lunch.

Lunch

--Large green salad

--Mock potato salad made with lightly steamed cauliflower, chopped carrot, onion, celery, and hard boiled eggs. Mixed with a dressing of Vegenaise, goat yogurt, mustard, celery seed, cayenne, apple cider vinegar, and honey.

Mock Potato Salad
(http://jireh.us/3-16)

I know many people love potato salad. Even though this doesn't use potatoes, it really does have a close resemblance to potato salad.

Snack

--Pumpkin seeds

--Goat cheese

Dinner

As I've mentioned before, we usually don't eat a large meal on Sunday evenings. We usually snack or have something light.

--I made us coconut shakes with coconut milk, eggs, vanilla extract, cinnamon, nutmeg, ice, and stevia.

Week 3 – Day 17 Results

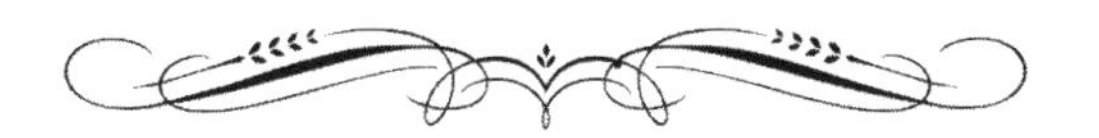

Two plus weeks ago, we began our AIEP (Anti-Inflammatory Eating Plan). I've read and studied various books and articles on inflammation by several different authors. I've taken what I believe to be the best information from several sources and devised a plan that I think is quite doable for anyone who is ready to take their health to the next level.

Here is what we ate on Day 17.

Breakfast

--Turkey bacon

--Eggs with peppers, onions, spinach, Herbamare, and cayenne

--We shared a fresh apricot and an apple.

Snack

--Pecans

Lunch

We actually ate later on in the day since it was a holiday. Jerry and I are NOT grill experts. Being vegetarian for many years, we didn't even own a grill until a few years ago, when we decided to join the 21st

century of American households and purchased a medium sized gas grill.
--We grilled chicken breasts and zucchini.
--We had leftover cauliflower "potato" salad on top of mixed greens.

Supper/Snack

I made us a treat. We have a small ice cream freezer that makes yummy treats. I wanted to see if I could make some ice cream and stay within the parameters of our current AIEP.
--I mixed coconut milk, eggs, vanilla, stevia, and a small amount of honey in the blender. I added slightly thawed, organic frozen strawberries, and blended again. I froze that mixture in the ice cream maker.
Since we've not had anything sweet other than fruit for nearly three weeks, this frozen dessert was delicious and plenty sweet. The strawberries, stevia, and small amount of honey gave it a great flavor. The coconut milk made it creamy. (And for those who don't care for the taste of coconut, you couldn't taste it. The strawberry flavor came through loud and clear.)

Week 3 – Day 18 Results

Here is what we ate on Day 18.

Breakfast

--We had a rather seedy breakfast. Flax seeds, hemp seeds, sesame seeds, sunflower seeds, Super Seed, vitamin C powder, almond butter, coconut milk, and blueberries. Very filling.

Lunch

--We had fresh vegetable juice made with fresh romaine lettuce, cucumber, parsley, celery, carrots, and a lemon.

--Then we snacked on goat cheese and fresh vegetables with almond butter.

Snack

--Apple,

--Almonds

Supper

--I made chicken salad with the leftover grilled chicken. I added celery, onion, walnuts, and an apple. Dressing was a mixture of Vegenaise, goat yogurt, Dijon mustard, curry powder, apple cider vinegar, and Herbamare.

Snack

--The yummy left over homemade strawberry ice cream.

Week 3 – Day 19 Results

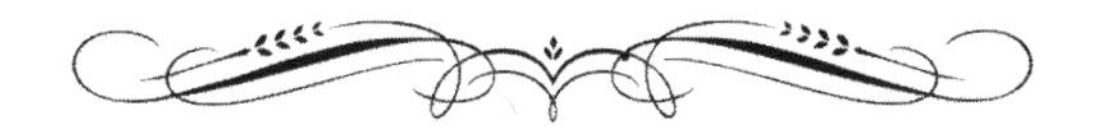

Here is what we ate on Day 19.

Breakfast

--We did our partial fast day. So, I made vegetable juice for us when we returned from the gym. I used fresh romaine and other fresh lettuce, celery, cucumber, and carrots.

Lunch

--I made us a green smoothie with spinach, zucchini, avocado, Nitro Greens, water, and ice. It was VERY green!

Supper

--I had broccoli and mushrooms that needed to be eaten. So, I made a casserole using steamed broccoli, sautéed mushrooms and onions and leftover turkey bacon. I made a sauce of Vegenaise, goat yogurt, eggs, goat cheese, spices, and herbs. Mixed the two together and topped it with chopped walnuts and sprinkled paprika on top. Baked it for about 35 minutes. It was quite good.

--We had a small spinach salad as well.

Broccoli Mushroom Casserole Photo
(http://jireh.us/3-19)

Snack

--Pumpkin seeds

Week 3 – Day 20 Results

To reiterate a bit, nearly three weeks ago, Jerry and I started on an anti-inflammatory eating plan. The purpose of the eating plan is to stabilize blood sugar levels, balance hormonal levels, and decrease inflammation in the body.

During the first two weeks we ate protein such as beef, chicken, and salmon. We ate eggs, non-starchy vegetables, and berries such as blackberries, blueberries, raspberries, and strawberries. We also ate lentils, almonds, walnuts, and other seeds. You'll notice that what we didn't eat was breads, pasta, rice, or potatoes. Nor did we eat any packaged, processed food.

After two weeks, we added more fruits, sweet potatoes, beans, and some different nuts. Still no breads, pasta, rice, or white potatoes. Again, the purpose is to decrease systemic inflammation in the body. Although Jerry and I eat a clean, healthy diet and have no real physical problems, we're doing this to remain healthy and to also come along side our readers should they want to eat a more healthful diet.

We'll go one more week with our current foods and then reevaluate where we go next. When we first began this eating plan, Jerry fell while working in the garage. He went down full force on his left arm on the concrete. Although his arm isn't broken, it was severely bruised and sprained. So, he's had limited mobility and also been in pain for the past several weeks.

I'm confident that eating the AIEP has helped with not only reducing inflammation in the arm but also helping to expedite the healing process in his arm.

We've also receive some interesting comments...all of which we appreciate. A few have commented that it didn't seem like we ate much protein or enough food in general and someone wondered why we were eating so MUCH protein. We're happy for each and every one of you who are reading our blogs and on this journey with us. Keep your comments coming.

Breakfast

--Smoothie made with coconut milk, spinach, eggs, Super Seed, and frozen mixed-berries

Snack

--Almonds

Lunch

--Leftover broccoli casserole

--Spinach salad with other fresh vegetables

Supper

--Wild-caught cod. I pan seared it with onions in coconut oil and then added some leftover organic pasta sauce that I had in the frig and wanted to use. It was very tasty.

--Baked sweet potatoes with butter
--Raw vegetable salad of cut up cucumber, onion, avocado, tomato and pepper, with olive oil and brown rice vinegar dressing

Wild-Caught Cod Dinner Photo
(http://jireh.us/3-20)

Week 3 – Day 21 Results

Here's what we ate for Day 21.

Breakfast

--Special birthday breakfast yesterday for my honey! I sautéed peppers, onions, and spinach in coconut oil and then added eggs and cooked them ever so slightly.

--Fresh mixed berries (strawberries, blueberries, blackberries, and raspberries) in a bowl with a spoonful of coconut milk, drizzle of honey, and sprinkle of cinnamon on top. Very pretty and very tasty.

Snack

--Blueberries

Lunch

--We snacked later in the afternoon with leftover salad from the night before.

--Jer ate some walnuts. I ate some blackberries.

Supper

Made a special dinner to celebrate Jerry's birthday.

--I never really buy steak...for several reasons. But I did splurge and bought the healthiest NY Strip Steak I

could find. Hormone and antibiotic-free, vegetarian-fed. Probably not grass-fed, but didn't have access to that and I wanted something special to celebrate.
--I gave the birthday boy a menu to choose from with various sides to go with the steak. He chose a green salad and baked sweet potatoes.
--I made him "angel-eggs" too. (Nothing that good should have the name "devil" in it.) Anyway, one of his favs.
--Of course he had to have a birthday dessert. I needed to get creative since we're not eating grains at the moment. I made a little cake with almond flour, arrowroot powder, eggs, coconut, stevia, butter, and vanilla extract. It was more like shortcake. I split each piece lengthwise, spooned mixed berries on top, added another layer of cake, more berries, and then drizzled whipped coconut milk overtop. Put a candle in it and sang, "Happy Birthday!"

Birthday Cake Photo
(http://jireh.us/3-21)

[Special note from Jerry -- Can you tell she loves me? She's a pretty awesome lady!]

Week 4 – Day 22 Results

Here's what we ate for Day 22.

Breakfast

--Sunflower seeds, sesame seeds, hemp seeds, almonds, almond butter, Super Seed, and OsoLean whey protein powder mixed with coconut milk and fresh berries.

Snack

--Walnuts and almonds

Lunch

We worked outside much of the day (90+ degrees) so we were very tired and lunch was very late.

--Large salad with fresh vegetables, goat cheese, sunflower seeds, and bacon

--"Birthday cake" with fresh berries

Large Vegetable Salad Photo
(http://jireh.us/4-22)

Supper

--Snacked on apples and almond butter

Week 4 – Day 23 Results

Here's what we ate for Day 23.

Breakfast

--Sunflower seeds, sesame seeds, walnuts, Super Seed, and OsoLean whey protein powder mixed with goat yogurt and fresh berries.

Snack

--Pecans

Lunch

--I cut up the leftover steak into strips and we dipped the strips in a sauce of Vegenaise, mustard, and wasabi powder (horseradish powder.)

--A large salad with fresh vegetables

--"Birthday cake" with fresh berries

Supper

--Snacked on cantaloupe and kiwi

--Apples and almond butter.

Week 4 – Day 24 Results

Here's what we ate for Day 24.

Breakfast

--Smoothie with coconut milk, spinach, eggs, frozen mixed berries, Super Seed, OsoLean Powder, and NitroGreens.

Snack

--Cantaloupe

Lunch

--Fresh marinated vegetables in olive oil and various vinegars, herbs, and spices. I used organic baby bella mushrooms, cucumber, pepper, tomatoes, avocado, and onion. Added chopped walnuts and

Marinated Vegetables Photo
(http://jireh.us/4-24)

stirred into salad. Served it on a bed of fresh spinach. (We're out of mixed greens.)

Snack

--Strawberries

Supper

--Hamburgers

--Black Bean Salad; I mixed rinsed and drained, canned black beans with chopped red pepper, celery, onion, garlic, parsley, and zucchini. I made a dressing of olive oil, Dijon mustard, tamari, fresh lemon juice, and brown rice vinegar. Poured it over salad along with chopped walnuts and mixed all together.

--Cantaloupe

We usually include beans often in our diet. However, I realized last night that when we eat beans it's in the form of soup or chili-type meal. In other words, I serve them hot. And lately it's been really hot here outside. So, my mind hasn't thought of hot dishes which included beans. I think more about salads, vegetables, and fruits with easy protein that doesn't require heating the oven or having the stove on for long periods of time. So, we've been eating cooler type foods and foods that are easier to prepare.

But beans are a great source of fiber and a good mixture of complex carbohydrates with protein. So, they're a nutrient dense food and very good for us to eat. And there are many ways to use them in the hot, summer months in various salads.

Week 4 – Day 25 Results

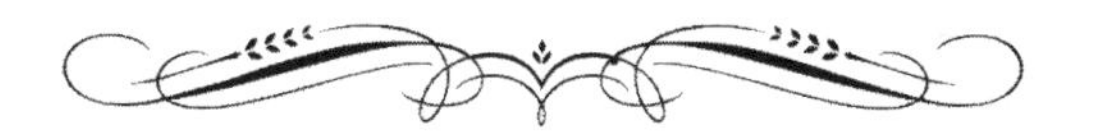

To reiterate a bit, a little over three weeks ago, Jerry and I started on an anti-inflammatory eating plan. The purpose of the eating plan is to stabilize blood sugar levels, balance hormonal levels, and decrease inflammation in the body. Watch this video (which is transcribed below) at:

Video of Results
(http://jireh.us/video)

In it I'll give you some insight to how it's going for us.

Video Transcription

"Hi! This is Sharon Graham, your health and wellness coach. If you've been following us lately, you know that we've been eating an anti-inflammatory eating plan.

"We began nearly four weeks ago with a plan designed to stabilize blood sugar levels, balance hormones, and decrease inflammation in the body. Now the premise of the eating plan is actually two-fold in that we're increasing the amount of nutrient-dense, mineral-rich foods that we're eating as well as eliminating food known to increase inflammation in the body.

"And even though we were eating healthy before, I have noticed that my desire for something sweet is gone. I no longer have any food cravings. Now we eat and enjoy our meals and we are satisfied. It seems like we're consuming less food and the tendency to overeat has been greatly diminished. Yes, we can overeat even the good stuff.

"Another positive benefit that I've noticed is the deep, sound sleep that I've been experiencing. I still might wake up to go to the bathroom because I drink so much water, but I immediately fall back to sleep and fall into a deep, sound sleep. I'll go to bed at 10:00, 10:30 at the latest, and I wake up at 6:00, 6:30 refreshed and ready to go.

"So just remember that you can read the list of foods that we've been eating, and you can follow the day-by-day menus that we've been eating by going to our Coaching Pair blog.
[www.TheCoachingPair.com/blog].

"And by the way, we would love to hear your feedback on what you've experienced if you've been following the anti-inflammatory eating plan." [End of Transcription]

Here's what we ate on Day 25. Wow! I never dreamed that I would post what I've eaten for all the world to see for 25 days. It seemed a bit daunting at the onset but like most things done over time, it's become a habit and is developing its own rhythm.

Breakfast

--Goat yogurt with fresh blueberries, strawberries, sunflower seeds, sesame seeds, almond butter, cinnamon, vanilla extract, and Super Seed

Lunch

--Leftover hamburgers, marinated vegetables, and black bean salad

Snack

--Goat cheese

Supper

--Salmon patties made with wild caught, canned salmon, chopped celery and onion, beaten egg, almond meal and cayenne pepper, pan seared in coconut oil.

--Yellow summer squash and onion stir fried in coconut oil. Seasoned with ground chipotle pepper and Herbamare.

--Coleslaw with red and green cabbage; Vegenaise, and apple cider vinegar dressing

Salmon Patties Photo
(http://jireh.us/4-25)

Our daughter knows her Daddy well. Part of his birthday gift from her and her family was a bottle of ground chipotle pepper. Actually, Jerry purposed to introduce her to "hot and spicy foods" when she was a little girl. And it stuck. Now, she's sending him some great smoky, ground hot pepper. It has such a wonderful aroma and really added flavor to the squash.

Week 4 – Day 26 Results

Last Saturday was the three-week mark for being on the anti-inflammatory eating plan. We'll go one more day eating the current foods and then re-evaluate where we go from here.

Here's what we ate on Day 26.

Breakfast

--Yesterday was our partial fast day. I made us vegetable juice using romaine lettuce, parsley, celery, cucumber, and carrots.

Lunch

--Green smoothie mixed in the blender with spinach, zucchini, parsley, NitroGreens, water, and ice.

Supper

--Leftover salmon patties

--Coleslaw

--Black Bean Salad

--Apple

Snack

--Sesame seeds, sunflower seeds, coconut, hemp seeds, almond butter, vanilla extract, coconut oil, and stevia mixed together; formed into small balls.

Week 4 – Day 27 Results

Here's what we ate on Day 27.
Breakfast
--Sautéed onions, peppers, and spinach in coconut oil with lightly cooked eggs.
--Kiwi and Clementines
Lunch
--I was running errands but before I ran out the door, I grabbed an apple and some pecans. I believe Jerry ate an apple, some carrots, and some goat cheese.
Snack
--Blueberries
Supper
--Lettuce wraps with free range turkey breast
--Mock potato salad made from cauliflower
--Strawberries

We are winding down on week four of the AIEP. It's been a great experience for both of us. Other similar eating plans would now begin to add whole grains such as quinoa, and brown rice along with whole grain/sprouted breads back into the diet. Other nuts such as cashews and pistachios can also now be included.

Other fruits such as bananas, papaya, and mango could also be added. Unsulfured dried fruits such as dates, figs, raisins, and prunes can also now be included. (I would have to say that if I have missed any foods on this plan, it's been dried cranberries. We really like them on our salads.)

Carob powder and an occasional treat of organic dark chocolate along with occasional organic red wine can also be added.

Jerry and I have chatted and have decided that with a few exceptions such as dried cranberries and occasional organic dark chocolate, we're going to stay with the second phase of the eating plan. We may on occasion eat some brown rice or quinoa, but we've decided for now that we won't return to eating the sourdough spelt bread and sprouted tortillas that we ate before.

So, I'll return to writing Daily Grams on other health-related issues, but I won't be continuing the running monologue about what we eat each day.

Thank you to all of you who have followed us, encouraged us, and sent in your comments. We appreciate each and every one of you!

Coach Sharon

May I Ask a Favor?

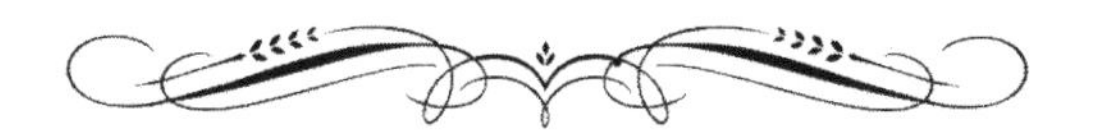

Thank you for watching over my shoulder as I describe our experience with the AIEP.

Now, may I ask a favor of you? I would love for you to leave a review on my Amazon page as your comments will assist others looking for information, and will assist me in the development of future books.

Simply go to:

www.amazon.com/dp/B007JOPN2U

Look for a button that reads "Create your own review" on the right side of the page and click the button to get started.

Thank you so very much.

Blessings to you!
Coach Sharon.

Meet the Author

Sharon Graham worked in the traditional medical field as a Registered Nurse for a number of years, and has over thirty years of experience in the natural health field as well. After being chemically poisoned in the mid-1980's, her immune system was nearly destroyed, resulting in a quest for answers apart from the traditional medical model.

That search led her into an intensive study of several complementary forms of health care. She has studied with the National Institute of Nutritional Education (now American Health Science University), and has taken many self-study courses in herbal medicine, homeopathy, and nutrition. She is a certified Life and Leadership Coach, a certified TLS Weight Loss Coach, and a certified Nutraceutical Consultant.

As a result of her personal journey to recover her own health, she has a desire and passion to educate and support others as they take responsibility for their own health. As a wellness, weight loss, and nutritional coach and consultant she brings a wealth of proven, practical information and methods so that you can achieve your own personal health goals. She has worked with hundreds of individuals to educate and support them in making lifestyle and nutritional changes, using both her traditional medical background as well as her knowledge of nutrition.

She has taught natural foods cooking classes and has given nutritional presentations to various groups of people. As a natural foods cook her clients say, “Sharon makes health food taste good.” She is also a blogger, is currently compiling a natural foods cookbook, and recently published a book on reducing inflammation in the body which is available from Amazon.

Disclaimers

Disclaimers / Legal Information: Copyright © 2012 by JIREH Marketing, Inc. All rights reserved. No part of this book may be reproduced, stored in a retrieval system or transmitted in any form or by any means, without the prior written permission of the author/publisher, JIREH Marketing, Inc.; 421 Currituck Drive, Chesapeake, VA, 23322, USA www.TheCoachingPair.com. The single exception is in the case of brief quotations for the purpose of writing critical articles or reviews.

Notice of Liability: The author and publisher have made every effort to ensure the accuracy of the information herein. However, the information contained in this book is presented without warranty, either express or implied.

Trademark Notice: Rather than indicating every occurrence of a trademarked name as such, this book uses the names only in an editorial fashion and to the benefit of the trademark owner with no intention of infringement of the trademark.

NOTES:

NOTES:

NOTES:

7079768R00053

Made in the USA
San Bernardino, CA
20 December 2013